Welcome!

Thank you for purchasing your copy of the Intuitive Health Workbook. To maximize your transformation, please fill out these worksheet as your read the corresponding chapters in the book, "Intuitive Health: transform yourself from the inside out."

Answer each question honestly and deeply. This is your journey. The more you embrace the experience and let go of your judgments, the greater your transformation will be. Use the journal pages to write down your thoughts and experiences as you add in each new action step. This is beginning of your transformation from the inside out.

AlliGardner.com

WHY HEALTH?

What does it mean to be healthy to you?

    Why health?

Do you meet your own definition of health?   O Yes   O No

    Why or Why not?

How will you feel when you are healthy?

How will you look when you are healthy?

How will being healthy affect your life?

How will being healthy affect those closest to you?

What do you feel is holding you back from being healthy?

How long have you been working to improve your health?

What has prevented you from improving your health?

Why do you want to improve your health?

Are you ready and willing to do whatever it takes to improve your health?

   O   Yes   O   No

Who Are You?

What was your childhood like? Describe your family and home life.

What did you do for fun? What activities?

What foods did you eat?

Were your parents or caregivers healthy?　　O　Yes　　O　No

　Were they active?　　O　Yes　　O　No

How did your parents or caregivers handle stress?

Did they exercise, turn to food, drink alcohol or smoke, yell?

Do you see any of these behaviors in your own life? If so, which ones?

How do you handle stress? How does it affect your life?

Does this bring up any behaviors that you would like to change?

If so, what are they?

Why do you want to change these behaviors?

How do these behaviors relate to your health?

Fears/Support Worksheet

How will your life improve when you achieve your goals?

Who will be affected by your achievement?

How will you feel if you don't achieve your goals?

How will those closest to you be affected if you don't achieve your goals?

What fears do you have around achieving your goals?

How will you overcome those fears?

What support do you need to achieve your goals?

Who will support you?

Why will you benefit from this support?

When will you ask for support?

Where will you receive support?

Limiting Belief Exercise

Write out fifteen beliefs that you have about nutrition, exercise, and health. Examples: "No pain. No gain." This is not true. You do not have to hurt to benefit from exercise. Healthy food tastes bad. Not true. You just haven't found what you like. Overtime your taste buds adjust as your eat whole, unprocessed foods. You body will crave what it needs. Exercise is boring. You haven't found that type you enjoy or you're ready for something new.

- ❧
- ❧
- ❧
- ❧
- ❧
- ❧
- ❧
- ❧
- ❧
- ❧
- ❧
- ❧
- ❧
- ❧
- ❧

Write down where you heard each belief. Is it something from your childhood or something you read or heard or something you know from experience?

Put and X through the beliefs that you know are not true.

Circle the beliefs that you question.

I encourage you to explore these beliefs.
Re-write a new list of YOUR beliefs about health, food, and exercise.

15 NEW Beliefs About Nutrition, Exercise, and Health.

∽

∽

∽

∽

∽

∽

∽

∽

∽

∽

∽

∽

∽

∽

∽

The Circle of Life

Discover which primary foods you are missing, and how to infuse joy and satisfaction into your life.

What does YOUR life look like?

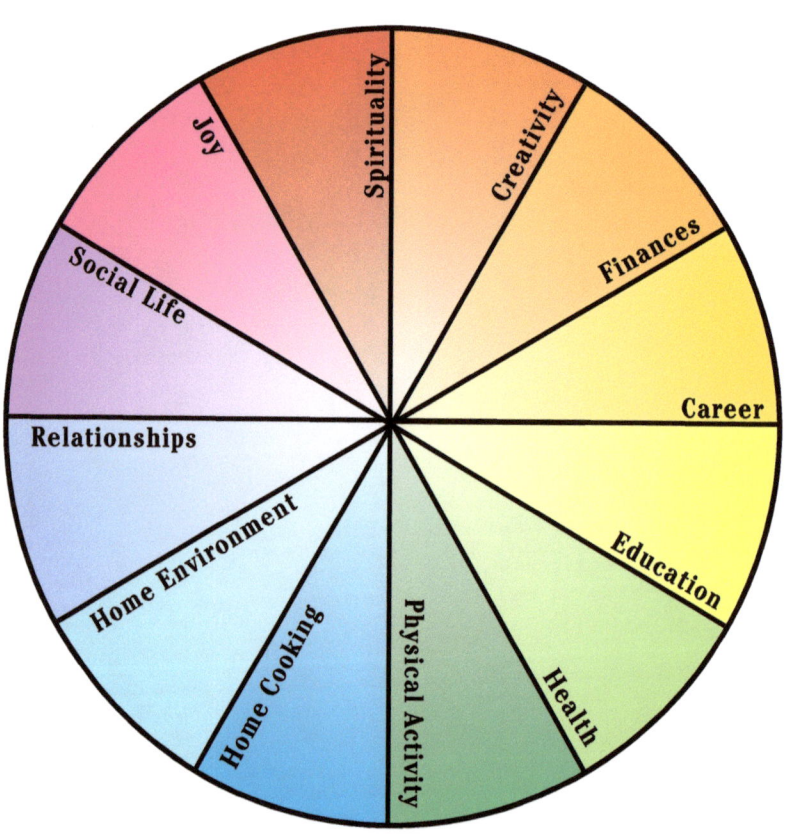

© 2015 Alli Gardner

1. Place a dot on the line in each category to indicate your level of satisfaction within each area. Place a dot at the center of the circle to indicate dissatisfaction, or on the periphery to indicate satisfaction. Most people fall somewhere in between.

2. Connect the dots to see your Circle of Life.

3. Identify imbalances. Determine where to spend more time and energy to create balance.

List your top 3 areas that need improvement.

    ∽

    ∽

    ∽

S.M.A.R.T. Goals Worksheet

Specific. Your goals must be specific and clearly defined.

Measurable. Your goals must be measurable.

Achievable. Your goals must be achievable.

Realistic. Your goals must be realistic.

Timely. Your goals must have a time component.

Examples of SMART goals:

"I will eat at least one serving of greens everyday in January."

"I will engage in physical activity for at least thirty minutes, five days each week."

"I will have date night with my significant other every other week."

"I will write in my gratitude journal five times each week"

As you write you goals, make sure to address

Primary and Secondary Foods.

6 Month Goals

❧

❧

❧

Three Month Goals

❧

❧

❧

One Month Goals

❧

❧

❧

Daily Habits Worksheet

Make a list of those things that you do almost every day, i.e. your morning routine.

Which habits are improving your health?

Identify which habits are detrimental to your health.

List three new healthy habits to implement this week.

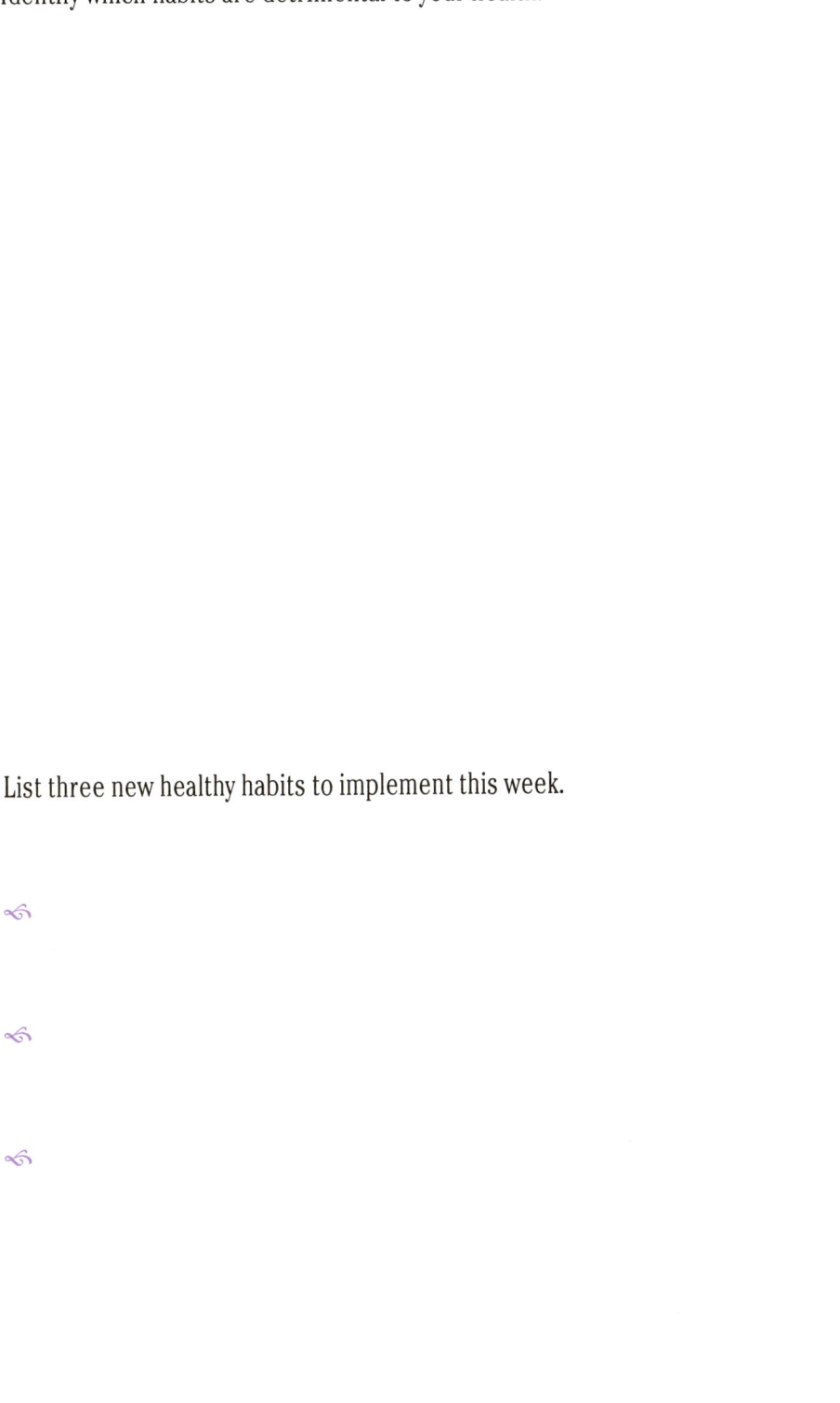

What Is Your Life Purpose?

Create a list of the top five things you value most in life. For instance: time for family, loyalty, honesty, health, integrity, freedom, activity, creating things, teamwork, independence, generosity, security, etc.

Which one do you value most?

What are you great at?

What things do you look forward to doing every day?

Name three things that come naturally and easily for you.

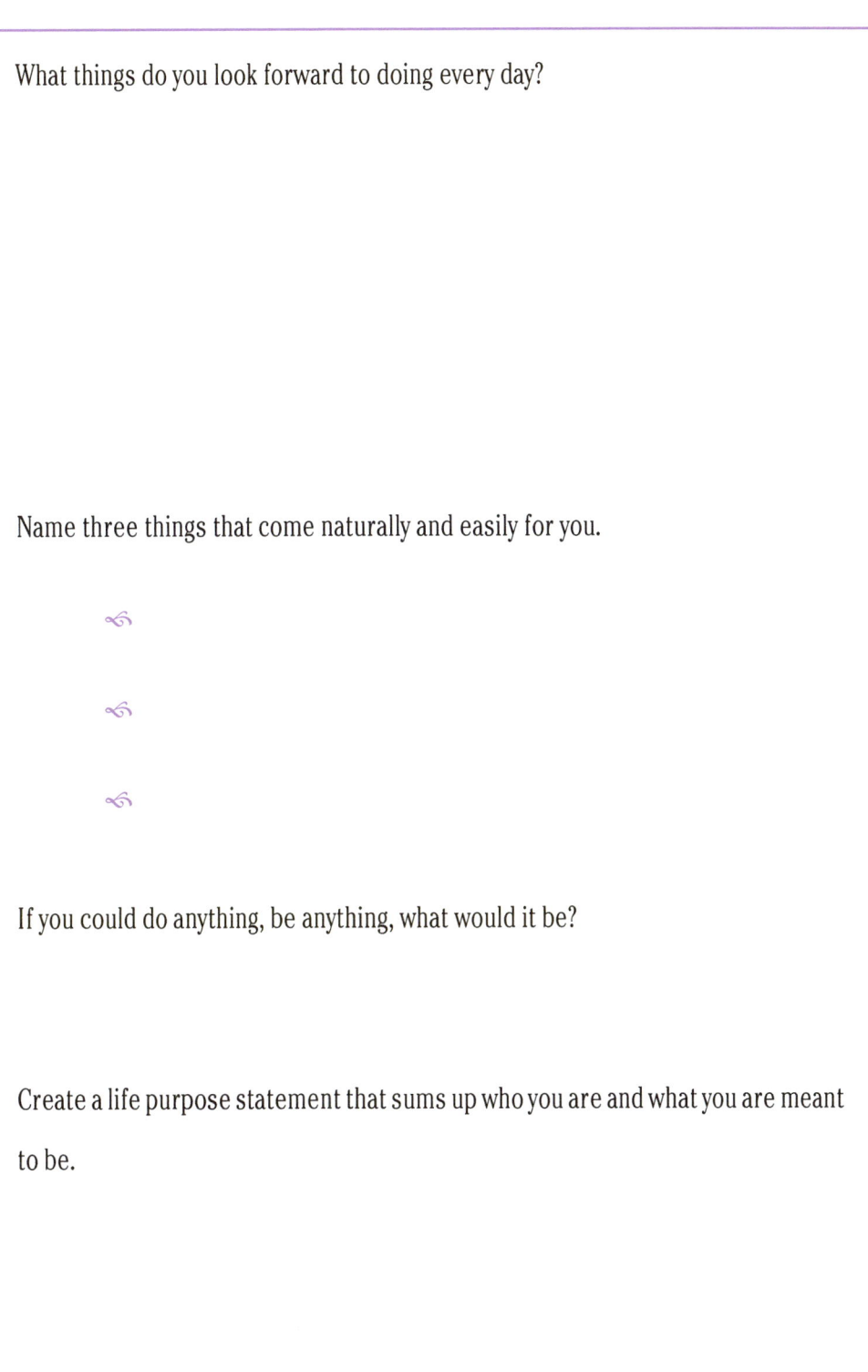

If you could do anything, be anything, what would it be?

Create a life purpose statement that sums up who you are and what you are meant to be.

Write down this statement and place it somewhere you can read it everyday.

Vision Exercise

Write out a detailed ten-year vision. Where do you see yourself in ten years? What is your ideal life? What if you have all of the resources, time, money, and support you need. What do you truly desire?

Next, keeping your ten-year vision in mind, **write out your three-year vision.** What things must happen in three years for you to be on track to reach your ten-year vision?

What do you need to achieve in the next year to be on track to achieve your three year and ten year visions?

Set 3 SMART Goals for **the next year**.

∽

∽

∽

Write down your goals and place them somewhere you can read them everyday."

My Nutrition Blueprint

A nutrition blueprint is a set of guidelines that you follow as you make food choices. It is not meant to be a set of hard and fast rules that you follow to a T. Make a list of guidelines you can strive for in making nutrition decisions.

For instance: I eat healthy meals 90% of the time, eat whole foods, avoid high fructose corn syrup, eat my favorite foods first.

❧

❧

❧

❧

❧

❧

❧

Over time your blueprint will change as you learn
more and your body adapts to eating healthy foods.

Self-Care Minimums

Read each question then spend two minutes writing. Do not stop writing for the entire two minutes. Leave the judgment behind and fill in the blanks. List whatever comes to mind.

Without _____ **I lose myself.**

When I feel most connected to my center I am _____ .

When I feel most connected to something larger than myself

I am _____ **.**

I can live without _____ **but not for long.**

Review your lists. Highlight the items that are repeated. These are your self-care minimums. These are the things that make you who you are and make you happy. Focus on these items to create a life that you love. Make these minimums a priority and incorporate them into your daily routines.

When you take care of yourself, you do everything else better.

Thoughts

Thoughts

Thoughts

Thoughts

Thoughts

Thoughts

Thoughts

Thoughts

Thoughts

Thoughts

Thoughts

Thoughts

please visit alligardner.com

subscribe to my newsletter for
more tips and information about
nutrition and healthy living

learn more about
additional products and
health coaching programs

contact me at
alli@alligardner.com

www.ingramcontent.com/pod-product-compliance
Lightning Source LLC
Chambersburg PA
CBHW050758290526
45792CB00008B/2233